From Broken to Strong

By

Bruno Laliberte

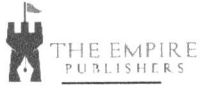

THE EMPIRE
PUBLISHERS

12808 West Airport Blvd Suite 270M Sugar Land, TX 77478,
Unites States

https://www.theempirepublishers.com/

Our books may be purchased in bulk for promotional,
educational, or business use.

**Please contact The Empire Publishers at +1 844 636-4579, or by
email at support@theempirepublishers.com**

First Edition December 2024

About the Author

Bruno Laliberte was born in Montreal and raised just north of the city in Laval. Though he left school during high school to start working, he always excelled in his studies. His academic success came easily, even without studying, but his passion for practical work and hands-on experience ultimately drew him out of the classroom and into the workforce.

With a career spanning both the food and golf industries, Bruno has spent most of his life navigating the fast-paced demands of the food business. Outside of work, he finds inspiration and peace in nature, often escaping to the woods for fishing trips or quad rides. These quiet, reflective moments in the wilderness offer a sharp contrast to his busy warehouse life and have become a key influence on his creative work.

One fun fact about Bruno is that, despite his size, he never had issues with bullies or troublemakers in school—or anywhere else, for that matter. It's a mystery that still amuses him, and he hopes to one day figure out why. Guided by his personal motto, "Be the smartest but let everyone think you're foolish," Bruno brings both humor and humility to his approach in life.

Currently, Bruno is working hard to achieve a significant milestone: securing a food certification for an upcoming project.

To his readers, Bruno encourages resilience and determination: "Try to stay strong, set some goals, and push and fight for them."

Acknowledgment

I would like to extend my heartfelt gratitude to The Empire Publishers for their unwavering support throughout this journey. A special thanks goes to Ned Harris, who believed in me and this project from the very start. I will always cherish the conversations we shared and the invaluable guidance he offered.

I am also deeply thankful to my friend and mentor, Michel, who has been a source of strength and encouragement through every step of this process, especially during challenging times after my separation. Michel, your belief in me and your mentorship, even before Juliette entered the picture, have left an indelible impact on my life. Thank you for everything you've done and for your faith in my abilities.

Dedication

This book is dedicated to anyone facing struggles after a breakup or during tough times in life. Remember, every hardship carries the potential for something beautiful and meaningful to follow. Let go, accept your circumstances, and keep moving forward. Set new goals for yourself and focus on them. Most importantly, strive to remain positive—it may seem difficult, but the transformation it can bring is truly life-changing.

Table of Contents

Chapter 1:
From Turf to Teeth

My life was pretty typical—work I adored, countless nights out with friends. I mean, who wants to stay cooped up in a small room all the time, right? But truth be told, I've always been a bit of a lone wolf. Don't get me wrong, I love my alone time too.

Born and raised in Quebec, we've got a hefty snowfall heading our way, about 20 to 25 centimeters. Sometimes, I wish I was born somewhere warmer. I can only imagine how lovely it must be.

As I sit here reminiscing, the memories flood back like a torrential downpour on a sun-drenched day. My life before seems like a distant echo of another reality.

I have always loved golf. But a decade ago, I was more than just a golfer; I was consumed by the game. Mornings were heralded by the crisp sound of club meeting ball, the dewy grass underfoot, and the promise of perfecting my swing. It wasn't just a weekend hobby; it was a daily ritual, a pilgrimage to the green sanctuary where I found solace and purpose.

Those early morning drives to the course, with the world still slumbering, were my sanctuary. The hum of the engine and the quiet anticipation of the day ahead were my companions as I charted my course through the day. Work was a means to an end, a necessary interruption in the pursuit of my passion.

And then there were the tournaments, where my dreams were forged and shattered. I still remember that Canadian tour qualifier. It still stings like a fresh wound. You see, I kind of missed the cut by a single shot. It was a solitary stroke that stood between me and destiny. But what can you do when fate is not your best friend? It was a bitter pill to swallow, knowing that one swing, one stroke, could have changed everything.

But as they say, everything happens for a reason. And perhaps that missed opportunity was the catalyst for a different journey, one that led me to… *her*. Yet, even in the warmth of her embrace, the echoes of the fairway beckon me back to a time when the only thing that mattered was the next hole.

Before *her*, there was Max - my friend, my confidant, my constant companion on the green. We were more than just friends; we were kindred spirits bound by our love for the game. From dawn till dusk, we traversed the course together, chasing that elusive **perfect** round.

Living under Max's roof was more than just a convenience; it was a home for two wandering souls united by a shared passion. His generosity knew no bounds. He offered me shelter in times when I needed the most. One always remembers such deeds of kindness.

And then there were the highs and lows, the peaks and valleys that defined those years. From surgeries to setbacks, each obstacle was just another hazard to navigate on the path to greatness. By surgeries, I actually mean a time when I had a collapsed lung – a pneumothorax they called it. It loomed there, threatening to derail my dreams, but even in the darkest moments, the green called out to me, offering hope where there seemed to be none.

As I lay on the operating table, the sterile scent of the hospital lingering in the air, I found myself grappling with the fragility of life. Yet, even as the surgeon's scalpel danced across my skin, I clung to the vision of fairways stretching out before me, promising redemption and renewal.

Recovering from the surgery was a grueling process, a test of both body and spirit. But with each labored breath and tentative step, I got better.

While golf was my main passion, there were plenty of other hobbies that added flavor to the mix.

I spent a lot of mornings by the water's edge, with nothing but the gentle lapping of waves and the promise of adventure. Fishing became my escape, a chance to unplug from the chaos and reconnect with nature's harmony.

Back in my younger days, I was a bit of a sports enthusiast. From the lightning-fast pace of badminton to the strategic finesse of ping pong and tennis, I dabbled in a bit of everything. Even hockey, with its icy showdowns and adrenaline-pumping action, held a special spot in my heart.

But amidst the whirlwind of activities, one thing remained constant - my pursuit of excellence. Whether I was on the golf course or the hockey rink, I poured my heart and soul into every game, driven by a hunger to push my limits and reach new heights.

Yet, beyond the thrill of competition, there was another side to my life that brought me immense joy - friendship. While Max was my partner-in-crime on the greens, he was just one piece of the puzzle. My social circle may have been small, but it was filled with people whose presence brightened my world in ways I never expected.

You know, it's funny, when someone asks about people who've made a difference in your life, you might expect family or friends to come up first. But for me, it was actually my boss, Michel. He's been a huge influence on me, both personally and professionally.

Back in the day, I had some dental issues. My teeth weren't exactly picture-perfect, you know? So when Michel hired me for the first time, he didn't just see a guy with crooked teeth. He saw potential. He gave me a position that involved dealing with a lot of people, and he didn't stop there. He actually talked to management and arranged financial help for me to fix my teeth. Can you believe that? It wasn't just about looks; he wanted me to feel confident and be successful in my role.

I underwent some serious dental work. It wasn't a walk in the park, but it wasn't as painful as I thought it would be. More nerve-wracking than anything else, really. But Michel and the team had my back throughout the whole process.

And you know what's even better? Michel and I are still very good friends to this day. He's moved up in the company, now he's VP, but our bond hasn't changed. We're still close, both personally and professionally.

When it comes to my job, that company was my big break. I started there when I was just 16, doing basic tasks like picking orders and driving a forklift. But over time, I moved up the ladder pretty quickly. Within a year or so, I was in a leadership role, overseeing the evening shift. It was a major growth for me, and I owe a lot of that to Michel's guidance and support.

In total, I spent almost 16 years at that company. Sure, I left for a while to pursue golf, but I ended up coming back. And even when I left again for a few years, Michel's influence stayed with me. He even hired a personal coach to help me develop professionally.

There's also another person who played a huge role in shaping who I am today: my high school teacher, Jean Pierre. Now, high school was a bit of a rough patch for me. I went from being a straight-A student to barely scraping by, and I even got kicked out of school for a bit.

But then came Jean Pierre in my life. He was like no other teacher I'd ever had. Instead of sticking to the usual rules, he gave us some freedom. We could wear hats, chew gum, even eat in class! But here's the catch: if we respected him and did our work, he didn't care about the rest.

It might seem like a small thing, but it made a huge difference. Suddenly, school wasn't just about following rules; it was about learning and growing together. And you know what? It worked. Jean Pierre got through to us in a way no other teacher had before.

When I think about the people who've left a lasting impact on my life, Michel and Jean Pierre are right up there at the top. They didn't just teach me lessons; they showed me what it means to be a mentor, a friend, and someone who truly cares about your success.

It's fascinating how life's trajectory can shift unexpectedly over time. Initially excelling academically in high school, my journey took an unforeseen turn during the second year, prompting a transfer to a different school. This new environment had a reputation for accommodating students who didn't conform to traditional norms, including individuals like myself.

It proved to be a formidable challenge. Instances of conflict were not uncommon, yet I found myself reluctant to engage in physical altercations. Instead, I assumed the role of an observer, preferring to remain hidden while others resolved disputes.

Though I occasionally tested the limits of acceptable behavior, there were certain principles to which I steadfastly adhered. Among them was a firm commitment to abstaining from physical confrontations. I wanted to avoid unnecessary conflicts at all cost. However, despite my best efforts to remain detached, there were moments when circumstances spiraled out of control.

There's this one memory that really sticks out in my mind — a time when things got way out of hand at school and ended with the police showing up at my house during dinner. It felt like something out of a movie, with the cops surprised that I, of all people, could be involved in a fight. It made me realize how unpredictable growing up can be.

Looking back on those school years, it's clear they were a mix of good and bad times. While high school had its tough moments, they also helped shape who I am today.

When I think about my past, there's this one moment that really stands out. It was a fight on the playground, me against a bully. Looking back, I feel proud of standing up for myself, even though I was usually the one getting picked on. It felt like a win, a rare time when I didn't back down.

At home, things were mostly good in the early years. Dad worked hard, Mom took care of things at home, and my brothers and I had fun together. But like any family, we had our arguments. I was always the serious one, not always seeing eye-to-eye with my more carefree brothers.

Growing up in that environment, I often felt like I didn't quite fit in. While my brothers jumped into things without thinking, I liked to watch and think things through. It made me different, even when I was young. Now, watching my daughters, I see a bit of myself in one of them—a quiet, thoughtful nature that reminds me of myself when I was young.

As time went on, our family faced some tough times. My mom's struggles with alcohol changed our happy home. Around thirteen or fourteen, I couldn't take it anymore and moved out to live with a friend for almost a year. It was a way to escape the chaos for a while.

Through it all, my brothers stuck around, dealing with things their own way. We never talked much about what was happening, but their support meant a lot. Eventually, my parents split up, marking the end of one chapter and the start of something new for us.

After the turbulence at home, my journey took a winding path. Leaving my parents' house at thirteen, I sought refuge with my father for a brief spell. By fifteen or sixteen, my parents' divorce marked a definitive shift. I moved in with a friend, then another, before finally carving out my own space in a small condo by the river.

During this period, I was also employed, finding stability in work amidst the chaos of personal life. It wasn't until later, after returning from a decade-long hiatus, that I reunited with Michel and found myself working with him once more. These transitions weren't easy, but I took baby steps ahead.

My life, as you read on, was not ordinary. But that's the best part about any story.

The words of a wise philosopher echoes in my ear: "Life is not about waiting for the storm to pass, but learning to dance in the rain." And boy did I dance.

Chapter 2:
Tug of Ambition

Warehouses have always held a strange appeal for me. Perhaps it's the controlled chaos, the constant activity, or the satisfying feeling of a perfectly packed order rolling out the door. But for me, it's more than just a workplace; it's a dance floor.

Life surely is a whole lot like a warehouse. There are days when things run smoothly, like a well-oiled machine. But then there are those downpours, those unexpected opportunities that come crashing down. That's when I grab my metaphorical umbrella and take a move. Because I don't believe in waiting for the sunshine. When it rains opportunity, I don't just stand there and get soaked. I grab an umbrella, turn up the music, and start dancing. It's about creating your own moves, your own rhythm, no matter the circumstances. It's a philosophy I've carried with me throughout my life, and it's made working in distribution centers a whole lot more successful than you might think.

My warehouse journey began with the most fundamental step – picking orders. I was like learning the art of finding the right products for customers. It was a solid foundation, but after a year, that familiar desire for growth started to startle me. I wanted the challenge, the responsibility. So, I took a leap and became the night shift supervisor.

Suddenly, I wasn't just the one picking orders; I was handling the entire night crew. It was a crash course in leadership, making sure orders were filled accurately, deadlines were met, and everyone on my team knew their steps. It was demanding, exhilarating, and I succeeded on the pressure.

Although this wasn't in my job description as a night shift supervisor, it pushes you beyond your comfort zone. It was during this time that I discovered a hidden passion – helping others learn and grow. I wasn't just a lone wolf, content with my own solo; I enjoyed the collaborative spirit, the conforming steps that come with a well-trained team.

A few years later, the warehouse implemented a new Warehouse Management System (WMS). The manager at the time resisted the new system with every fiber of his being. But I saw it as an opportunity to improve our efficiency and flow. So, I dug in, learned the WMS inside and out, and even helped train the Toronto staff on its implementation. This is where I truly learned the art of warehouse management – the subtle balance between efficiency, accuracy, and team morale. Through it all, I learned that a good manager is more than just a boss; they're a conductor, keeping the warehouse in perfect working state.

My warehouse career wasn't without its challenges. There were times when the music felt monotonous, the steps repetitive. There was a period where I felt the need to explore new fields. So, I took a chance on a career in golf course retail. While it wasn't the perfect fit, it gave me valuable experience in purchasing and negotiation – skills I could translate back to distribution centers.

Moreover, people management wasn't always my forte. As a night shift supervisor, the focus was on tasks and deadlines. But over time, I discovered the value of developing my team. I found myself enjoying mentoring new hires and helping them grow in their roles. It became a key part of my leadership philosophy.

No doubt, there are always challenges in people management. Personalities clash, and sometimes motivation wanes. But the rewards far outweigh the struggles. Seeing a team member grasp a new concept, overcome a hurdle, or simply take ownership of their role – that's what makes it all worthwhile.

However, when I was back, when Michel called me, I was once again into this warehouse job. But after some period of time, we faced a problem: the work was more and more and I needed an assistant. Beyond that, the ever-present challenge of warehouse management – finding the right people – became even more crucial.

There is no denying that interviewing can be a bit of a gamble. You only have a short time to assess someone's potential. But I had my key ingredients in mind.

First and foremost, I needed someone who wasn't afraid to learn. Technical skills could be taught, but a genuine hunger for knowledge was essential. A candidate who asked thoughtful questions and showed curiosity to learn.

Teamwork was another crucial ingredient. Warehouses are a work of moving parts, and everyone needs to play their part in harmony. So, I looked for people with strong communication skills, people who could collaborate and help their teammates win because a happy team is a productive team.

So, with my list of must-have qualities in hand, I started on the interview process. Resumes piled up on my desk.

And then, we met them. Two individuals who stood out from the rest: Michelle and Juliette. Both possessed potential, but their strengths lay in very different areas.

Michelle walked in with an air of quiet confidence, her resume telling years of experience. Juliette, on the other hand, exuded a different kind of energy. While her experience wasn't as extensive as Michelle's, there was a spark in her eyes, a genuine curiosity that drew me in.

"Juliette," I began, "you might not have as many years under your belt, but your resume highlights some impressive skills in data analysis. How do you see yourself using those in a warehouse setting?"

Juliette's face lit up. "Absolutely! I believe data can be a powerful tool for identifying inefficiencies. For example, I could analyze pick times to see if there are areas where workflow could be optimized."

Her answer surprised me. It wasn't the typical response I received. Here was someone who saw beyond the daily tasks and looked for ways to improve the entire system. It was a fresh perspective, one that spoke volumes about her analytical skills and her forward-thinking approach.

The interviews continued, each revealing more about the candidates. Ultimately, the "dancing in the rain" philosophy came into play. I needed someone who wasn't just qualified, but who could adapt to the ever-changing environment of the warehouse. In Juliette's eyes, I saw a hunger for knowledge, a willingness to learn and grow alongside the team. She was the perfect complement to the existing crew.

Perhaps the most compelling aspect of Juliette's candidacy was the sense of partnership I felt. She wasn't just looking for a job; she was looking for an opportunity to learn, to contribute, to be a part of something bigger. There was a spark of collaboration in her, a willingness to work alongside the existing team, to share her knowledge and learn from theirs. That, in itself, was a valuable asset.

In the end, it wasn't just about her skills or her experience. It was about the potential for growth, for collaboration, for creating a future where the warehouse wasn't just a workplace, but a platform for innovation and shared success. Juliette, with her enthusiasm, her analytical mind, and her collaborative spirit, was the perfect candidate.

The decision was made. Juliette would be joining the team, and together, ready to face whatever challenges the next day threw at us.

With Juliette on board, there was the crucial task of integration. I didn't want to just throw her into the deep end of the warehouse; I wanted her to feel welcome, supported, and ready to contribute her to the team.

Chapter 3: Juliette's Arrival

Now, let me tell you about the day Juliette joined our warehouse crew. It was a bright morning, the kind that sets your bones right after a long winter. Juliette walked in, a touch of nervousness in her eyes. I gave her a big smile, enough to light up the whole place, and said, "Welcome aboard, Juliette! Let's show you the ropes around this warehouse of ours!"

Our warehouse was something else entirely. Shelves stacked high as a church steeple, filled with more boxes than you could shake a stick at. Workers scurried around, moving things with those fancy forklift machines that beeped and blinked like fireflies in the night. It was a sight to behold, that's for sure.

Our first stop was my office, a little corner nook where I kept track of all the orders coming in and going out. It wasn't much to look at, just a desk and a computer screen that buzzed all day long. But for Juliette, it was going to be her own little command center, where she'd make sense of all the comings and goings.

Then, we ventured deeper into the heart of the operation. The picking area was a real beehive of activity. Men and women, armed with scanners and carts, weaved through the shelves like a well-oiled machine. Juliette watched with wide eyes, taking it all in like a sponge.

"This is where the magic happens," I said, pointing towards the warehouse area. "Orders come in, and these people find all the bits and bends the customers need."

She gave a small nod, a smile tugging at the corners of her lips. "It's like a puzzle, isn't it?" she said, her voice full of wonder. "Seems chaotic at first, but there's a way to it all."

Now, you have to understand, it wasn't all smooth sailing. New places can be overwhelming like a sudden downpour. There were new words to learn, like "SKU" and "backstock," and the constant buzz could be a lot for someone not used to it. But Juliette, bless her heart, was a quick learner. She asked questions, good ones too, and soaked up information like a parched field drinking in the rain.

Of course, there were some hesitations. But as time passed, the warehouse felt peaceful, like the calm before a summer storm. Maybe it was because things were a bit slower than usual, or maybe it was the way we all worked together, like parts of a big clock. Whatever it was, it was a perfect introduction for Juliette, a chance to ease into the rhythm before the real work began.

As the day wore on, things picked up again, and Juliette dove headfirst into her new job. Her fresh perspective, like a breath of spring air, was a welcome change. And as we navigated the warehouse together, I knew deep down that Juliette wasn't just here to learn. She was here to add a new verse to our warehouse song, a verse filled with new ideas and ways of doing things.

The next target was integrating Juliette into the team: it was a breeze, truth be told. Now, I'll admit, I had a sliver of concern at first. We had a good number of people on the team with disabilities, and Juliette, well, she had a strong personality. But then again, she was a realtor in her past life, and those ones should be good with people, right? That's what I figured anyway. Working with people who have disabilities is a whole different ball game, though. So, there I was, a tiny knot of worry in my gut.

But those worries flew out the window faster than a feather in a hurricane. Everyone took to her right away. Even today, they still ask about her, how she's doing, a testament to the kind of connection she made. It was like a perfect match.

Now, about assigning tasks – I definitely played to her strengths. At the beginning, it was more specific duties, but eventually, she graduated to a bit of everything. Think of it like a chef's apprentice, learning the ropes one dish at a time.

In the early days, her main focus was this program we had for the marketing and sales teams. They'd put in orders for custom builds, and Juliette had to be the guardian of deadlines. She'd pore over the data, making sure everything got pulled and built on time. Think of her as a conductor, ensuring the whole warehouse orchestra played in perfect harmony.

That was just the first act, though. I also tasked her with creating a brand new seller sheet, a fancy term for a report that tracked a bunch of things we hadn't before. This one kept tabs on labor costs, how long tasks took, and the bottom line – were we making money or losing it? Let's just say Juliette shed some light on areas where we could tighten our belts.

And that brings us to the real magic: how Juliette's spirit impacted the team. Like I said, everyone warmed up to her. The transition from me being the go-to person to her being the new expert was smooth as butter. It freed me up a bunch, and seeing the team take to her so easily put a genuine smile on my face. Juliette wasn't just a good worker; she was a great teammate, someone who made the whole warehouse feel a little more like a family.

Juliette's arrival was a godsend when it came to data analysis. Now, when I rebuilt the division, I did it the best way I knew how, but let's just say spreadsheets weren't exactly my forte. Building those beautiful, intricate reports, the kind that make data sing, well, that was where Juliette shone.

She also had an eye for patterns, a way of dissecting complex data sets and turning them into stories we could all understand. She'd point out trends I'd missed, ask insightful questions that forced me to re-evaluate things. She'd often pull out actionable insights that helped us work smarter, not harder. Take the team structure, for example. I thought I had it optimized, but Juliette's analysis revealed some hidden inefficiencies. We adjusted the team setup based on her findings, and the results were immediate. Productivity soared, bottlenecks vanished, and orders started flowing through the warehouse like a well-oiled machine. It was a work of efficiency, all thanks to Juliette's ability to translate the numbers into a language of improvement.

And the improvements weren't just internal. We started hitting deadlines consistently, which previously felt like chasing a mirage. Our clients were happy, our team morale was high, and it all stemmed back to Juliette's data-driven approach.

Here's a memory that always warms my heart. Just a few months after Juliette joined us, there was this annual gala hosted by the agency that connected companies with disabled employees. We won the award for "Best Company" that year, and I clearly remember Juliette by my side, smiling with pride. It was evidence of the positive impact she'd made, not just on our bottom line but on the lives of the very people we were there to support. That night, under the lights of the gala, it wasn't just an award we celebrated, it was the dawning of a new era for our warehouse, an era fueled by data, collaboration, and the quiet brilliance of Juliette.

If you want to know, how Juliette's impact on warehouse efficiency was undeniable, then let us look into it. Within a few short months, the place was humming with a newfound productivity. The late orders, those missed deadlines, became a thing of the past. Before her, my days were a constant scramble. Late projects piled up, my inbox overflowed, and keeping track of everything felt like an impossible feat. Juggling sales, operations, marketing, and a struggling warehouse division – it was a recipe for chaos. But Juliette's data analysis skills cut through the clutter. She identified bottlenecks, pinpointed inefficiencies, and most importantly, presented solutions backed by hard data. Suddenly, we weren't just guessing; we were making informed decisions that yielded measurable results. The metrics we used to track performance – the Key

Performance Indicators, or KPIs – told the whole story. Order fulfillment times plummeted. Accuracy rates soared. We weren't just meeting deadlines; we were exceeding them. The warehouse, once a source of frustration, became a well-oiled machine, a testament to Juliette's organizational skills and data-driven approach.

And it wasn't just about crunching numbers. Juliette also streamlined workflows with innovative ideas. She replaced the homegrown order system with a new system that seamlessly integrated with our existing infrastructure. It was a game-changer, providing real-time order updates and ensuring everyone was on the same page.

Another key improvement stemmed from Juliette's communication skills. She took the lead in liaising with marketing and product management teams. New promotions, upcoming launches – she ensured everyone in the warehouse was in the loop, prepared for any changes that might impact order fulfillment. There were no more surprises, no more scrambling at the last minute. Her approach wasn't about micromanaging; it was about clear, honest communication. She built trust with these teams, ensuring that nothing fell through the cracks. Information flowed freely, and the warehouse became a truly collaborative environment.

Along with these skills, what appeared most interesting to me was her personality and her interactions with the team, especially those with disabilities. Let me assure you, sympathy wasn't something I needed to teach her. She possessed a natural calm and patience that resonated with everyone. She'd take the extra time to explain things clearly, to break down tasks into manageable steps. It wasn't just about efficiency; it was about genuine care and understanding.

The bigger challenge, surprisingly, came from some of the long-time employees. People who'd been there for fifteen, twenty years, set in their ways. Change, even positive change, can be met with resistance. Introducing new ideas, especially from a newcomer, could be met with a silent "not invented here" attitude. Juliette confronted those waters with grace, though. She presented her ideas with data, with logic, and a genuine respect for the established systems. It wasn't about tearing things down; it was about building something better, together.

There were stumbles along the way, of course, but Juliette's perseverance, coupled with her ability to connect with people, ultimately won over even the most skeptical team members. In the end, everyone benefitted from her fresh perspective, and the warehouse thrived under her influence. It was a true indeed demonstration of the power of mentorship, of learning from each other, and of embracing change for the better.

To be honest, my initial expectations for Juliette were fairly straightforward. I needed someone to handle the office paperwork, the endless follow-ups, the administrative tasks that kept me tethered to my desk. But Juliette surprised me in the best way possible. Sure, she mastered those tasks, but she also craved the energy of the warehouse floor. She wanted to see things in action, to understand the flow of work firsthand.

So, I gave her the freedom to explore. I let her shadow pickers, chat with forklift drivers, and delve deeper into the daily life of the warehouse. It was a revelation. Her understanding of the big-picture data was amplified by this ground-level perspective. She could see where the data pointed to inefficiencies, but now she also understood the human element, the reasons behind some of the bottlenecks.

I must say that she exceeded my expectations in a way I could never have predicted. She wasn't just a data expert; she was a bridge between the numbers and the people who made them sing. And in doing so, she not only improved the warehouse's efficiency, but also my own approach to management. It was a lesson in humility, a reminder that sometimes the best way forward is to listen, learn, and adapt.

One more thing I should tell you, though it may appear as If I am praising myself but that is not the case. I am just showing reality. And the fact is that I definitely do see myself as a mentor to Juliette in a way. We worked together at SID Foods for a year and a half, and even after that, our paths crossed a few times. I guess you could say I played a part in launching her into a whole new career path. And it is true that mentoring Juliette was a unique experience. She came from a completely different world – real estate, but here she was, diving headfirst into the fast-paced chaos of a warehouse. It was a lot to take in, and for the first few months, it was understandable that she held back a bit, still finding her footing.

But then, Juliette's strong personality, the one I initially worried about, started to shine in a positive way. She wasn't afraid to ask questions, even the tough ones that challenged the status quo. This warehouse had been running a certain way for a long time, and Juliette's fresh perspective was a breath of innovation. That's when the mentoring dynamic truly kicked in. I spent a lot of time teaching her the particulars of warehouse management, the unspoken rules, the political scenario of a big company. There's a certain finesse needed to pass through those waters, and I wanted to make sure she had the tools to succeed.

Moving further, if you ask, how Juliette's arrival improved me in the context of work, then the answer is this: Her arrival forced me to take a long, hard look at my own management style. After years in the warehouse, you get comfortable in your routines. You develop a way of doing things, and it becomes gospel. You might listen to suggestions, but sometimes that listening has a built-in filter – a filter that murmurs, "Hey, this is how we've always done it, and it works just fine." But Juliette shattered that filter. Her data-driven approach, those insightful questions that poked holes in my assumptions – it was a wake-up call. I started listening more, truly listening, not just to her, but to everyone on the team. New ideas, once dismissed as "untested" or "too risky," were suddenly met with an open mind. It was a humbling realization, but a necessary one. The warehouse wasn't a one-man show, and my way wasn't always the best way. Juliette, with her fresh perspective, showed me the value of collaboration, of harnessing the collective wisdom of the team.

Moreover, her arrival was also a game-changer for my workload and stress levels. Gone were the days of me being buried under paperwork. Follow-ups, orders, the endless administrative tasks – Juliette took them all on with a smile, freeing me up to focus on the bigger picture. Finally, I was able to step away from the desk and actually walk the warehouse floor. Suddenly, I had the time to observe, to strategize, to tackle projects that had been languishing on my ever-growing to-do list. The constant pressure of juggling a million tasks at once? It started to melt away.

One such project involved negotiating a new cardboard deal. This was no small feat – gathering quotes, comparing prices, negotiating terms. It was a time-consuming process, but with Juliette handling the day-to-day operations, I could finally dedicate the focus this project demanded. My mind was clear, my stress levels down, and I could finally close a deal that saved the company a significant amount of money.

As time passed, Juliette's impact went beyond just alleviating my workload. Her arrival sparked a wave of long-term ideas for the warehouse's future, and for her evolving role within the team. Freed from the daily grind, I could finally start thinking strategically. There were a couple of mandates I'd been given that, frankly, felt like dead ends without some serious help. One such project involved revamping the entire warehouse layout. The current setup was a maze of walls and inefficient workstations – a productivity nightmare. But before Juliette, tackling a project this size felt insurmountable. There simply weren't enough hours in the day.

And with Juliette at the helm, the picture changed entirely. Once she was settled in and comfortable, we started brainstorming. I redesigned the entire flow of the warehouse, optimizing workstation placement, maximizing storage space, and creating a layout that facilitated smoother workflow. It was a transformation, and it wouldn't have been possible without Juliette's arrival.

It is very true what people say about intermingling of people if they spend enough time together. And in the case of ours, I would say Juliette's influence wasn't confined to the warehouse walls. It spilled over into my personal life in a way I hadn't anticipated. Being able to delegate tasks, to trust her with the day-to-day operations, finally allowed me to achieve a semblance of work-life balance.

Gone were the 60, 65-hour workweeks. Suddenly, a 50-hour week felt like a luxury. Don't get me wrong, 50 hours is still a significant chunk of time, but it was a world of difference. Those extra hours meant evenings spent with family, weekends free for hobbies, and a chance to finally recharge. It was a simple thing, truly, but it made a world of difference in my overall well-being.

And this newfound balance had a ripple effect. Working with Juliette changed my approach to problem-solving. Remember, my old style was a bit…well, stubborn. I listened, yes, but sometimes that listening was filtered through a lens of "this is how we've always done it." But Juliette challenged that. Her questions, her data-driven insights, forced me to truly listen, to consider new perspectives. Suddenly, problem-solving became a collaborative effort. We'd bounce ideas off each other, dissect challenges from different angles, and ultimately reach solutions that were stronger, more innovative, and more sustainable. It was a refreshing change, and one that I continue to value to this day.

Everyone says that stress and constant pressure are slow poisons. In this context, if I had given another year or two of that frantic pace, I wouldn't be telling you this story. Burnout, health problems, maybe even a career change – who knows where that path would have led? But Juliette's arrival was a lifeline. She shouldered the burden of the day-to-day operations, freeing me from the constant firefighting. Suddenly, I had the clarity to breathe, to think strategically, to finally achieve that elusive work-life balance.

And this newfound balance wasn't just about leisure time. It allowed me to rediscover the joy of work itself. With less stress clouding my judgment, I could focus on the bigger picture, on making meaningful improvements to the warehouse. It was a return to the passion that had drawn me to this job in the first place. There was a sense of accomplishment, a shared success that resonated throughout the team. We weren't just colleagues anymore; we were collaborators, working together to achieve a common goal. And that, in itself, was a reward.

So, why was hiring Juliette a life-changing decision? Because her arrival wasn't just about spreadsheets and warehouse efficiency. It was about a transformation, both personal and professional. It was about learning to delegate, to trust, and to listen. It was about rediscovering the importance of work-life balance and the power of collaboration. And while my social circle might not have exploded overnight, the friendships I had became richer, more meaningful.

Chapter 4: Crossing the Line

I'd always prided myself on being a rational man. Logic and efficiency were my guiding stars, the principles I lived by. The warehouse, with its predictable paces and measurable results, was my domain. But then Juliette came along, and everything changed.

Initially, she was just another employee, albeit a particularly capable one. But as we spent more time together, side by side, walking through the complexities of the warehouse, a different picture began to emerge. I started to see beyond the sharp suits and polished demeanor.

There was a strength in her, a quiet determination that was both charming and inspiring. Her mind worked like a machine, processing information and solving problems with an efficiency that bordered on the uncanny. It was like watching a chess grandmaster anticipate every move. I found myself watching her, not just as her boss, but with a growing fascination.

And then there was her laugh. It was infectious, a warm, bubbly sound that could brighten even the gloomiest of days. It was in those shared moments of laughter, the easy banter, that I began to see a side of her that no spreadsheet or report could reveal.

It was as if I was discovering a hidden world, a world that existed beneath the professional facade. The more I learned about her, the more intrigued I became.

As I told above, my world had always been governed by a strict set of rules. Logic reigned supreme, emotions were kept in check. Dating an employee was a clear violation of this code. Not only was it against company policy, but it also felt like a breach of professional ethics.

As her boss, I held a position of authority. A romantic relationship would inevitably blur those lines, creating a power dynamic that felt inherently wrong. The potential for conflict of interest was a constant worry. Would my judgment be clouded? Could I truly be fair in my evaluations?

And then there was the fear of gossip, of becoming the subject of office chatter. I prided myself on my reputation as a level-headed, professional manager. A workplace romance could jeopardize that image.

The internal conflict was intense. On the one hand, there was the undeniable attraction, the spark between us that grew stronger with each passing day. On the other, there were the potential consequences – both professional and personal. It was a battle between heart and head, a struggle to reconcile the man I was with the man I was becoming.

Before this, for years, I had embraced the solitary life. The freedom, the independence, the absence of compromise – it was a lifestyle I had cultivated with care. There were no demanding partners, no children to chauffeur, no dinners to plan. My life was an accurately ordered puzzle, where every piece fit perfectly into place.

And yet, there was a growing sense of emptiness, a quiet acknowledgment that something was missing. I had convinced myself that this was enough, that fulfillment could be found in career success and personal hobbies. But as the years passed, a nagging doubt crept in. Was this truly all there was?

Juliette disrupted this carefully constructed existence. Her presence brought an effervescence, a spontaneity that was foreign to my world. In her company, I discovered a capacity for laughter and joy that I hadn't experienced in years. It was as if she had unlocked a part of me that had been dormant.

And then there was that night. The warehouse was bathed in the soft glow of the setting sun, casting long, dramatic shadows. Juliette had come to show her boyfriend her new workspace. She wore a red dress that seemed to ignite the room, and for a moment, I was breathless. There was something about her that evening – a confidence, a sensuality that was utterly captivating. It was as if a switch had been flipped, and I saw her in a completely new light.

That night, a seed was planted, a seed of desire and longing. I couldn't explain it, couldn't rationalize it. It was simply there, a force that pulled me towards her. And as the days turned into weeks, that seed grew into something stronger, something that challenged the carefully constructed walls of my solitary existence.

Hence, here I was. But being on the line between our professional and personal lives was like walking a tightrope. We both knew the risks, but the pull of our connection was undeniable. We were careful, at first, to keep our growing feelings under wraps. We'd steal glances across the warehouse, share knowing smiles, and find ways to connect without drawing too much attention.

But as our bond deepened, it became harder to hide. There were those stolen moments, like when we'd be working late and the rest of the office had cleared out. We'd find ourselves drawn to the same coffee machine, our conversations drifting from work to something more personal. It was in those quiet, stolen moments that our connection truly blossomed.

Of course, the office grapevine is a relentless force. Whispers started, and before we knew it, the whole warehouse was abuzz with speculation. People love a good story, and a boss-employee romance was juicy gossip. It was embarrassing, to be honest. I felt like I was betraying the trust of my team, and I hated the way it made Juliette feel.

It was at the company summer party that things really spiraled out of control. One minute we were laughing and enjoying ourselves, the next we were the center of attention. Someone had overheard us talking about weekend plans, and the rumor mill went into overdrive. It was as if a spotlight had been turned on us, exposing our secret to the entire office.

The memory of Juliette in that red dress, animated and electrifying, stayed with me long after her boyfriend walked her out of the warehouse that night. It was a turning point, a crack in the carefully constructed wall I'd built around my heart. I knew I had to act on this unexpected spark, but how?

There were a million reasons to play it safe. Company policy, the potential awkwardness at work… but the thought of burying this feeling, of letting this chance slip away, was unbearable. So, I decided to test the waters, to see if there was any spark beyond the professional.

A few weeks later, after Juliette had broken things off with her boyfriend, a group of us from the office planned a casual after-work drink. It felt like the perfect opportunity. I extended the invitation to Juliette, my heart pounding a little faster than usual. To my delight, she readily agreed.

The bar was buzzing with after-work energy, but my focus was solely on Juliette. She seemed different that night, less guarded, more relaxed. Maybe it was the absence of her boyfriend, or maybe it was just the atmosphere. Whatever it was, I found myself captivated by her every word, every laugh.

When the bar started to wind down, a couple of my colleagues suggested another spot to continue the night. It felt like the right moment to make my move. As we walked, the city lights painting a shimmering backdrop, I caught Juliette's eye.

"This place has a great rooftop bar," I said, trying to sound casual. "Care to join me for one more?"

A smile played on her lips. "Sure," she replied, the single word sending a jolt of excitement through me.

The rooftop bar was a world away from the noisy pub. The city stretched out before us, a glittering drapery of light. We found a quiet corner table, the only sound the soft murmur of conversation and the clinking of glasses.

As the night deepened, our conversation flowed effortlessly. We talked about work, about our lives, about our dreams. There was a spark there, an undeniable connection. I could feel it in the way her eyes held mine, in the way her laughter seemed to fill the entire space.

But I was hesitant. The memory of the drinks and the late hour held me back. Finally, after a shared glance that lingered a beat too long, I took a deep breath.

"This has been a great night, Juliette," I said, my voice a little rough. "I… I'd like to see you again sometime, if you're interested."

There was a flicker of surprise in her eyes, but it was quickly replaced by a warm smile. "I'd like that, Bruno," she replied, her voice soft yet firm.

It wasn't a grand declaration of love, but in that simple exchange, a doorway opened. We had taken the first step, a tentative exploration of the feelings simmering beneath the surface. And as we walked back to the hotel, the city lights seemed to shimmer brighter, reflecting the newfound hope that bloomed in my chest.

Discretion was our watchword in those early days. While the spark between us was undeniable, the complications of a boss-employee relationship were a constant concern. We couldn't risk jeopardizing Juliette's career or creating a hostile work environment.

So, we played a careful game. Stolen glances across the warehouse floor, hushed conversations during breaks – these were the breadcrumbs we left behind, clues that only the most observant might notice. There was a thrill in the secrecy, a sense of forbidden adventure that only intensified our connection.

However, keeping a lid on a blossoming romance wasn't easy. Sharing a laugh, a knowing smile – these were natural reactions that sometimes betrayed our carefully constructed facade. One of my closest colleagues, Michel, a man with an uncanny ability to read people, picked up on the subtle shifts in our dynamic. He didn't pry, but there was a knowing glint in his eyes whenever he caught us exchanging a private joke.

Later, we confided in a couple of other trusted colleagues, people who wouldn't spread rumors or gossip. It was a relief to share our secret with someone outside our immediate circle, someone who could offer support and a listening ear. But for the most part, the world outside our stolen moments remained blissfully unaware.

We knew, of course, that this secrecy couldn't last forever. The longer our relationship progressed, the harder it would be to hide. But for a while, the thrill of the clandestine, the shared burden of a secret, fueled the fire of our connection. We lived in a world of stolen glances and whispered promises, a fragile bubble of intimacy waiting for the inevitable moment it would burst.

My head and my heart were locked in a fierce battle. Here I was, Bruno, the ever-pragmatic manager, suddenly contemplating a relationship that could jeopardize everything I'd built. Logic screamed at me to walk away. The potential consequences were dire – a scandal in the office, a possible reprimand, even the kiss of death for my career.

The company policy on fraternization was clear. Upward mobility was within reach, and a messy workplace romance could derail everything. "Focus on the promotion, Bruno," a voice echoed in my head. "Don't let emotions cloud your judgment."

But then there was Juliette. Every interaction with her, every shared laugh, every stolen glance, chipped away at my carefully constructed walls. She was unlike anyone I'd ever met – intelligent, driven, with a spark that ignited a fire within me. The thought of losing her, of letting this connection slip through my fingers, was unbearable.

"Maybe it's worth the risk," a different voice whispered. "Life is too short to play it safe all the time." The potential benefits were intoxicating. The chance to share a life with someone who truly understood me, who challenged me, who made me laugh – it was a prospect I couldn't ignore.

This internal conflict wore on me. Sleepless nights were spent wrestling with the what-ifs. One evening, unable to bear the weight of the secret any longer, I confided in Michel. His unwavering support was a balm to my soul. He saw the spark between Juliette and me, and unlike the voice of caution in my head, he encouraged me to explore it.

Confiding in Michel was a turning point. The weight of the secret lifted a little, replaced by a newfound clarity. As I spoke, the fear of losing Juliette overshadowed all other concerns. Even the potential threat to my career seemed insignificant compared to the prospect of a life without her.

Then came the opportunity for a promotion, a chance to lead another division within the company. It was a pivotal moment. Taking it would mean leaving the warehouse, leaving the space where our connection blossomed. But it could also be a fresh start, a way to distance ourselves from the potential office drama.

"I don't care about the promotion," I confessed to Michel, my voice surprisingly steady. "I want to be with her, Michel. Even if it means leaving this company."

Michel, ever the pragmatist, raised an eyebrow. "Leaving might be a bit drastic, Bruno," he said with a knowing smile. "There might be other options."

And he was right. The promotion to another division, a fresh start within the same company, suddenly presented itself as a viable solution. It wouldn't be defying the rules as blatantly as leaving altogether, but it would create distance, a shield from the prying eyes and gossiping tongues of the warehouse.

More importantly, it would give us a chance to explore this connection outside the confines of work. We wouldn't have to steal glances or hold hushed conversations anymore. We could be open, honest, and truly see where this path might lead.

The decision was made. I applied for the promotion, driven not just by ambition, but by the hope of a future with Juliette. The interview process was a blur, fueled by nervous excitement. And then, the news arrived. I had the job.

The promotion was a bittersweet victory. On the one hand, it represented a step forward in my career. On the other, it meant leaving the familiar space where our connection had blossomed. But the prospect of starting anew, of building a life with Juliette outside the watchful eyes of the office, filled me with a sense of optimism that I hadn't felt in years.

Looking back, it seems obvious now. Taking the promotion wasn't just about career advancement; it was about creating space for our relationship to grow. It was a calculated move, a gamble fueled by the hope that the spark between us wouldn't be extinguished by distance. And deep down, I knew that if this connection was meant to be, it would survive anything, even the challenges of a professional separation.

Chapter 5: Nature's Magic

When I first pulled up to Juliette's home, I wasn't sure what to expect. I'd only ever known her through our work, where she was always professional, efficient, and somewhat guarded. But the moment I stepped out of my car and took in the scene before me, I realized I was about to see a side of her that she didn't show to just anyone.

Her home was remote, nestled in a quiet corner of the countryside, far removed from the bustle of city life. It was a big, sturdy house, yet there was something peaceful about it, like it had been standing there forever, a silent guardian of the surrounding nature. The air was thick with the scent of pine and earth, and the only sounds were the distant calls of birds and the rustling of leaves in the breeze. This wasn't just a place where Juliette lived; it was a reflection of who she was, a part of her that she had carefully cultivated, much like the garden that sprawled in front of the house.

I rang the doorbell, but there was no answer. Not surprised, I decided to walk around the house to see if I could find her. As I rounded the corner, I caught sight of her in the yard, and the sight stopped me in my tracks. Juliette was standing there, almost knee-deep in horse manure, laughing as she tried to clean up after one of the horses. Her hair was a wild mess, her clothes stained with dirt, but she was glowing with a kind of happiness I hadn't seen in her before. I chuckled to myself, thinking, "She's the one." In that moment, I realized that there was so much more to her than I had ever imagined.

Her connection to nature was evident in everything she did. I watched as she interacted with the horses, her touch gentle and reassuring, her voice soft yet firm. It was clear that she knew them well, understood their moods, their quirks. She moved with a kind of grace that only comes from years of practice, and I couldn't help but admire her even more. When she finally noticed me, she waved me over, a big smile on her face.

"Sorry about the mess," she said, laughing as she wiped her hands on her jeans. "These guys can be a handful sometimes."

"Don't worry about it," I replied, smiling back. "I think it suits you."

After she finished up with the horses, she suggested we go for a hike. I was more than happy to oblige. As we walked, the conversation flowed easily between us, and I found myself opening up to her in a way I hadn't before. The hike was challenging, but the views were worth it. We climbed higher and higher until we reached a ridge that overlooked a vast expanse of forest. The sun was beginning to set, casting a golden glow over the landscape, and for a moment, we just stood there in silence, taking it all in.

"This is my favorite spot," Juliette said softly, her voice filled with a kind of reverence. "Whenever I need to clear my head, I come here."

I nodded, understanding exactly what she meant. There was something about being out in nature, away from the noise and chaos of everyday life, that brought a sense of peace and clarity. As we stood there, I felt a deep connection to her, one that went beyond words. It was as if we were two sides of the same coin, both of us drawn to the quiet beauty of the natural world.

The hike back was almost as magical as the way up. We got a little lost at one point, which led to a lot of laughing and teasing as we tried to find our way. But even in that moment of uncertainty, there was a sense of ease between us, a comfort in each other's presence. By the time we made it back to the house, the sun had set, and the sky was a deep shade of indigo, dotted with stars.

That night, Juliette cooked us dinner, and I was struck by how at home I felt in her space. The house was warm and inviting, with a lived-in feel that spoke of years of memories and moments shared. Her mother and stepfather were away, so it was just the two of us in the bachelor suite downstairs, which only added to the sense of intimacy. The meal was simple but delicious, made with fresh ingredients from her garden. We talked about everything and nothing, our conversation flowing as easily as the wine in our glasses.

After dinner, we sat by the fire with a good whisky, and it was then that I realized how much we had in common. We shared a love of nature, of course, but there was more to it than that. We both appreciated the simple things in life, the quiet moments, the beauty in the ordinary. It was a connection that I hadn't felt in a long time, and it made me think about my own life, about the choices I had made and the path I was on.

Spending time with Juliette in her world gave me a new perspective on my own life. I had been alone for so long, focused on my career, on achieving my goals, that I hadn't stopped to think about what I really wanted. But the more time I spent with her, the more I realized that maybe there was something missing, something that I had been too afraid to admit to myself. I found myself thinking about the future, about what it would be like to build a life with someone who understood me in a way that no one else did.

The weekend flew by, and before I knew it, it was time to leave. As I packed up my things, I couldn't shake the feeling that something had shifted between us, that our relationship had deepened in a way that neither of us had expected. There were no grand declarations, no promises made, but there was a quiet understanding, a mutual respect that spoke volumes.

As I drove away, I found myself replaying the moments of the weekend in my mind. The way Juliette had looked at me when she thought I wasn't paying attention, the sound of her laughter as we stumbled through the woods, the warmth of her hand in mine as we sat by the fire. They were small moments, but they were the kind that stick with you, the kind that make you wonder what could be.

I knew that I was at a crossroads, that the decisions I made in the coming days and weeks would shape the rest of my life. But for the first time in a long time, I wasn't afraid. Juliette had shown me a different way of living, one that was slower, more intentional, more in tune with the world around us. And as I drove away from her home, I knew that I wanted to be a part of that world, that I wanted to build something real, something lasting, with her.

The weekend at Juliette's had been a revelation. It had given me a glimpse into a life that I had never considered before, one that was filled with love, laughter, and the quiet beauty of nature. And as I turned onto the highway and headed back to the city, I couldn't help but smile, knowing that whatever happened next, I was ready for it.

Chapter 6:
Love's Winter

As life moved ahead, the winter of change settled in slowly, much like the snow that blanketed Quebec in those early months. Juliette and I found ourselves with new roles, both at work and at home, and though the adjustment wasn't easy, it was something we took on together. My transfer to another division and her move into a new role within the company marked a significant shift in our lives.

It wasn't easy at the beginning. There was a sense of uncertainty at first, as we wondered how this change would impact our relationship. Juliette and I had been working so well together, almost seamlessly, and then everything changed. I thought the distance might strain us, but surprisingly, it didn't. I continued to coach her in her new role, guiding her through the challenges as best as I could. We were still close, still connected, and honestly, nothing really changed between us—except that we no longer worried about people finding out about our relationship. That fear, that constant need to keep everything under wraps, was gone, and it felt liberating.

When we rented our first house together, it was a new chapter in our lives. Moving in with someone is a big step, and we both knew it would come with its challenges. We divided the household tasks right down the middle—each of us taking on what we had to do. We worked well together, just like we had at the office. But things shifted when we bought our own home. Suddenly, the stakes were higher. It wasn't just about keeping a rented space tidy; it was about building a life together, laying down roots, and making decisions that would shape our future.

Living in Quebec didn't require much adaptation for either of us. This place is in our blood—it's all we've ever known. The cold, the snow, the long winters—it's just part of life here. But living together brought new dynamics to our relationship. I began to see different sides of Juliette, parts of her I hadn't fully appreciated before. Her organizational skills at work were impressive, but seeing her bring that same level of detail and structure to our home was something else. It wasn't what I expected, but it was a welcome surprise. And then there was the spiritual side of her, something I hadn't really noticed before. She was so grounded, so connected to something bigger than just the day-to-day grind. It was inspiring and deepened my admiration for her.

We didn't have a lot of time to find new hobbies or shared interests in our new environment. Everything happened so fast. Juliette got pregnant not even a year after we moved in together, and that brought its own set of challenges. There were complications with the pregnancy that kept us on edge, and then, about a year later, we bought our house. It felt like life was moving at breakneck speed, and we were just trying to keep up. But in the midst of all that chaos, we found our little moments together—quiet, simple moments that reminded us of why we chose each other in the first place.

Our friends and family were incredibly supportive during this time. I'd been alone for so long before Juliette came into my life, and they saw how happy she made me. They were happy for us too. But as time went on, something shifted. I couldn't quite put my finger on it at first, but there was a change in how they interacted with us. It wasn't until a few months later that I began to understand why, but that's a story for another time.

During this period, we both had our own career aspirations. Juliette was determined to grow in her role, to understand the ins and outs of operations. I did my best to coach her through it, to share what I knew, and to help her navigate the challenges. Today, she's a warehouse manager, and I'd like to think I played a part in her success. As for me, I was aiming for a director position. I left before I could make that happen, but now, after being back for almost nine months, I'm on track to reach that goal within the next year or so.

Like any couple, we had our share of disagreements. For the most part, we didn't argue much, but when we did, it was almost always about money. At that time, Juliette was making significantly less than I was, and that disparity was a big source of stress for her. It wasn't an easy thing to navigate, but we managed. We talked through it, made compromises, and found ways to support each other.

We started discussing long-term plans about six months after we moved in together. I was 42 at the time and wasn't entirely sure about having kids, but I knew that Juliette was the one I wanted to spend the rest of my life with. So, I went for it, and I'm happy I made that decision. Our plan was to live in the bachelor apartment at her mother's place to save money. But then her mother separated from her husband, and we ended up buying out his share of the house. It wasn't what we had originally planned, but it worked out for the best.

Living together taught me a lot about myself, about what I wanted in life, and about the importance of family. I had almost lost sight of that before Juliette came along. She brought me back to a place where I could see clearly again, where I could appreciate the simple joys of being loved and loving someone in return. It also made me more disciplined at home. I wasn't always the most organized person, but living with Juliette, I learned the value of keeping things in order, of creating a space where we could both feel comfortable and at peace.

In the end, this chapter of our lives, this "Love's Winter," as I like to call it, was about more than just surviving the cold or adjusting to new roles. It was about growth—both as individuals and as a couple. It was about facing challenges together and coming out stronger on the other side. And most importantly, it was about love—the kind that endures, that supports, and that transforms you in ways you never expected.

Chapter 7:
Territory Marked

Life has a funny way of shifting when you least expect it. Juliette and I had always found comfort in our routines, in the rhythm we had built together. There was a kind of quiet peace in the way we'd end our evenings, her head on my chest as we lay on the couch, the faint sound of music filling the air. Sometimes we'd talk about the future in vague, broad strokes—places we wanted to visit, dreams we had for our careers, and those wistful "what if" conversations that seemed harmless at the time. The idea of a family had always been there, lingering in the background, but never something we discussed with urgency. It felt distant, like a concept for "someday."

But life doesn't wait for you to be ready. It moves, and sometimes it hits you with a force that changes everything in an instant. Our plans, our sense of normalcy, were all about to be upended in ways we couldn't fully anticipate. I remember those days leading up to the change vividly. Everything felt the same, and yet there was an undercurrent, something unspoken building between us. Juliette had been a little more tired than usual, a bit quieter, though she insisted it was nothing. But I knew her better than that. Something was different.

Then, one evening, as the soft glow of the setting sun filtered through the windows, Juliette looked at me with an expression I couldn't quite read. There was a seriousness in her eyes, mixed with a glimmer of something else — was it joy? Fear? I couldn't tell. She took a breath, then said the words that would reshape everything: "I'm pregnant."

Juliette's words hung in the air for a moment, soft but loaded with meaning. Her voice was trembling with equal parts joy and fear.

The world seemed to tilt. My chest swelled with happiness, but there was an underlying current of worry, too. I had hoped for this moment, but the reality of it hit me harder than I expected. All those late nights we spent talking about our future and trying to conceive — they'd all led to this. The joy was immediate and overwhelming, but alongside it was a flicker of doubt, insecurity even. Were we ready for this? Could we handle it, especially financially? I had no idea what was coming, but the thought of becoming a father sent a shiver down my spine.

The first few days after finding out were blissful. We didn't talk about the logistics or the money much, at least not right away. I think we both wanted to savor the happiness, to let ourselves feel like everything was going to be perfect. There were still so many questions, though. How would this change our lives? What kind of parents would we be? I kept circling back to the same worries — how would we manage? But every time the doubt surfaced, I'd push it away. I wanted to focus on the joy, to stay in that space where everything felt possible.

Juliette handled it differently. From the start, she seemed to settle into her role as a mother-to-be effortlessly. Of course, at first, things didn't change much for us. We kept up our routines, our jobs, the daily grind. But slowly, I found myself taking on more tasks, more responsibilities. It was never anything we talked about directly; it just happened. She needed more rest, and I wanted to make things easier for her, so I started doing more around the house without even thinking about it. Our roles shifted naturally, but nothing felt burdensome. If anything, it made me feel more connected to her, more committed to our shared future.

Emotionally, I tried my best to be there for her, though I know there were moments when my own worries got in the way. Whenever she seemed unsure or anxious, I would remind her that we were going to be great parents, that everything would go smoothly. Sometimes I said it more for myself than for her, just to make the fear go away. But she seemed to take comfort in it, and I held onto that. I remember rubbing her belly every night, massaging oil into her skin. She loved that. It became our ritual, something that made the pregnancy feel more real and grounded. As her belly grew, so did our bond. I could see her body changing, and with it, her spirit, her energy. I couldn't help but fall in love with her all over again.

It wasn't long before the conversations turned serious. We talked about our future, what life would look like with a child. Marriage wasn't something either of us had been particularly interested in before, but as the pregnancy progressed, I began to reconsider. I didn't tell her at first. I wasn't even sure I was ready for that step myself. But I kept thinking about it, especially toward the end of the pregnancy. It felt like the right thing to do, like a way to mark this new chapter in our lives. I hadn't made any concrete plans, but the idea was there, sitting in the back of my mind, waiting for the right moment.

Then came the complications. It started with small warnings from the doctors. Juliette had some tests done, and the results weren't what we had hoped for. There were signs that something might be wrong with the baby, though they couldn't say for sure what it was. I tried to stay strong for her, but inside, I was a wreck. Juliette, though — she was the positive one. She kept reassuring me that everything would be okay, that our little girl would be fine. She was so calm, so confident, even when the doctors began suggesting that we consider ending the pregnancy.

Those were some of the hardest conversations I've ever had. Juliette made it clear that she wanted to continue, no matter what. But she left the final decision to me. It was one of the most terrifying moments of my life. I felt the weight of that choice in every bone, every muscle in my body. What if I made the wrong decision? What if our baby suffered because of it? I spent sleepless nights thinking about it, weighing the options. But in the end, I chose to continue. I didn't know what the future held, but I couldn't imagine not giving our child a chance.

Looking back, I'm so grateful for that decision. It brought Juliette and me closer than we had ever been. We had to lean on each other in ways we hadn't before, learning to trust each other's instincts, to be strong together. There were nights when we stayed up talking, not just about the baby but about everything — our fears, our dreams, our hopes for the future. It was hard, but it was also beautiful in its own way. We became a team, more than ever before. It felt like we could face anything as long as we had each other.

Our families were thrilled when we first shared the news of the pregnancy. There were tears, congratulations, and endless offers of support. But when the complications surfaced, things changed. People didn't know what to say or how to act, and I think that's when Juliette and I really leaned into each other. We had support from our friends and family, especially when they learned there might be a problem with our little girl, but in those private moments, it was just us. We had to rely on each other, and that made all the difference.

As the due date got closer, my emotions were all over the place. I was excited, of course, but also scared out of my mind. The doctors still couldn't tell us for sure what our baby's condition would be. They said she could be severely handicapped, or she could be born with no issues at all. The uncertainty was agonizing. I didn't know what to expect, and that uncertainty was the hardest part. I felt powerless, like I was standing on the edge of a cliff, waiting for the ground to give way beneath me.

The day of the birth arrived, and everything happened so fast. I didn't know I'd be able to assist in the delivery, but when the moment came, I jumped in. I was there, right by Juliette's side, holding her hand, watching as our daughter came into the world. My heart pounded in my chest, and for a split second, I forgot to breathe. Then she was there, tiny and perfect. I'll never forget that moment, the rush of relief and joy. We had made it. Our little girl was here.

She was born on May 28, 2020, right in the middle of the pandemic. The hospital was on lockdown, and we were stuck in that room for days, just the three of us. It felt surreal, like the rest of the world had faded away, and all that mattered was us and this tiny new life we had created. The complications, the fear, the uncertainty — it all seemed to melt away as I held her for the first time. She was healthy. She was perfect. And in that moment, I knew that everything we had gone through was worth it.

Becoming a parent changed everything for me. Before, I was living day to day, not really thinking about the future. But now, everything was different. I had someone else to think about, someone who depended on me. It was a life-changing event, no doubt about it. Every decision, every thought was now filtered through the lens of parenthood. It was scary, sure, but it was also the most fulfilling thing I had ever experienced.

As I sat there, cradling our daughter in my arms, I looked over at Juliette. She was exhausted but glowing, a smile on her face that told me everything I needed to know. We had made it. We had faced the unknown together, and we had come out stronger on the other side. Our territory had been marked, not just by the challenges we had faced but by the love and commitment we had for each other. This was the beginning of something new, something bigger than both of us. And I was ready for it.

Chapter 8:
Adverse Reaction

When my daughter was born, we felt an overwhelming mix of emotions. Joy, of course, but also fear—something dark and gnawing at the edges of our minds. The doctors had warned us early on, long before the delivery, about the genetic issue. It wasn't something simple or easily fixable. One of her chromosomes was missing a part, and another had an extra. They couldn't predict exactly how it would manifest. The specialists gave us two possibilities—she could be severely handicapped, or there could be no noticeable effects at all. And yet, despite the uncertainty, they were sure of one thing: they strongly recommended ending the pregnancy.

I remember that moment vividly. The room felt cold, sterile, even though Juliette and I sat together, holding hands, like we always did in those appointments. The doctor's words echoed in my ears. *End the pregnancy*. They left the decision in our hands, but it didn't feel like a choice—more like a command wrapped in white coats and clinical terms. I looked at Juliette, waiting for her to say something, to make sense of it all. But she was silent. When she finally spoke, her voice was steady, almost calm. "It's your decision," she said quietly. "I'll support whatever you choose."

That put me in a position I never thought I'd find myself in—a decision that could change everything. I knew, deep down, that if I told her to stop the pregnancy, she would've walked away, not just from the doctor's office but from me. I didn't want to lose her; I couldn't. But more than that, I couldn't bear the idea of losing our baby either, even if we had no idea what was waiting for us on the other side of those nine months. So, I chose to stay on this path, even though fear gripped me tighter with every passing day.

We coped with the unknown as best we could. There were nights I couldn't sleep, staring at the ceiling while Juliette lay peacefully beside me, convinced everything would be fine. Her belief in our daughter's future was unshakeable, and I leaned on that faith like a lifeline. I had to stay positive, if not for myself, then for her, and for the little life growing inside her. It wasn't easy, though. The fear didn't go away; it just hid under the surface, waiting for the quiet moments when it could creep back in. But we held onto each other. We became closer in ways I never imagined. Our conversations shifted—less about the "what-ifs" and more about "when" she arrives, what kind of parents we would be, and how we would face whatever challenges came.

Family and friends were supportive, offering words of comfort and encouragement, but the reality was, this was something Juliette and I had to go through together. No one could make the decision for us, and no one could carry the weight of it. I appreciated their kindness, but after a while, it became clear that nothing anyone said could change the situation. It was just the two of us, moving forward, step by step.

The real challenge, though, came two years later. By then, our daughter had grown into a quiet, sweet toddler, but she had always been slower than other kids. She wasn't walking or talking yet, and we were prepared for that. We knew her development would be different, but we loved her just the same. Then one day, out of nowhere, she fell from her chair. I can still hear the sound of her head hitting the floor—a sharp thud that made my heart stop. We rushed her to the emergency room, terrified, but after a scan, they told us she was fine and sent us home.

Relief washed over us, and we went back to our routine, grateful that it hadn't been worse. But that relief was short-lived. A few days later, her pediatrician called. He had just returned from vacation and reviewed her scan. I'll never forget the panic in his voice as he spoke to Juliette. I had just walked in from work, and she was pacing the house, frantic. "You need to take her to the children's hospital immediately," he told us. It turned out she had water in her brain, and if it had gone untreated any longer, we could have lost her.

The fear I had tried to push down for so long came rushing back, hitting me with full force. There was no room for doubt anymore; we had to act. The next day, she underwent surgery. I don't think I've ever felt so helpless in my life. I stood there, watching the doctors wheel her away, and all I could do was hold onto Juliette's hand, both of us trying to stay strong for each other. The hours dragged on, but when they finally brought her back to us, the relief was indescribable. She had made it through.

Juliette and I stayed strong through it all, but it wasn't because we weren't scared. We were terrified. But Juliette's unwavering belief that everything would be fine kept me going. I didn't always feel hopeful, but I had to support her, to mirror her optimism even when my mind was racing with worst-case scenarios. There were moments when I felt like I was pretending, acting the part of the confident father, when inside I was filled with doubt. But looking back, I realize that maybe that's what strength really is—choosing to believe in a better outcome, even when fear is screaming in your ear.

Our youngest daughter had just started walking by then, and as she grew, we did our best to shield her from the stress. But as she became more aware, it was impossible to hide everything. I think she sensed, even at a young age, that her older sister needed help. There was a bond between them that went beyond typical sibling rivalry. In a strange way, our younger daughter's milestones—her first steps, her first words—became a catalyst for her older sister.

But overall, the birth of our younger daughter brought a welcome sense of normalcy to our lives, even in the midst of the chaos. I remember her first steps, how early they came, and the way she quickly found her voice. She was always so eager, so full of life, and it was as if her natural growth and curiosity were beacons of light during an otherwise uncertain time. She didn't realize it, but every new milestone she hit filled us with joy—small moments that kept us anchored to something good, something normal.

We made a conscious effort not to let our focus on the older one overshadow the younger. It wasn't easy. The demands of the oldest daughter's health were always pressing, and we had to spend so much time ensuring she was getting the care she needed. But our younger girl—she wouldn't be left behind. She was always at my side, especially when I was working in the garage. She'd follow me around, pretending to help, her tiny hands clutching at tools far too big for her, but always determined to be part of it.

Some of my fondest memories are of us sitting on the tractor, cutting grass together. She loved it, sitting on my lap, holding the wheel, her face bright with excitement. It wasn't just the joy of her presence that made those moments special, though—it was the way she brought lightness back into our lives. In the midst of hospital visits, surgeries, and the constant worry over our older daughter, our younger one was like a breath of fresh air, a reminder that not everything had to be heavy and overwhelming. She gave us laughter when we needed it most.

Looking back, those moments taught me more about life than I ever could've imagined. If there was one thing I learned through all of this, it was that family is everything. It's the one thing that stands strong, even when everything else feels like it's crumbling. Family isn't just about love— it's about sacrifice, loyalty, and sometimes the sheer will to stay together when the weight of the world feels like it's too much to bear.

Juliette and I both knew that, no matter what happened, we would always love our children unconditionally, *forever*. That knowledge bound us together tightly during those first years. But as our younger daughter grew, something began to change. It's hard to say exactly when or why it happened, but the closeness Juliette and I once had started to fade. It wasn't a dramatic shift, nothing we could point to and say,

"This is where things went wrong." It was more like a slow drift, a gradual distance that crept in over time.

At first, everything we did was about surviving those early years together, staying strong for our daughters. But once the youngest was about a year old, things began to shift. It wasn't that we stopped caring about each other—we just stopped being as close. Maybe it was the stress of it all catching up with us, or maybe we had grown so used to being strong for our daughters that we forgot how to be strong for each other. I'm still not sure what caused it, but I know we weren't the same as we once were.

Despite the changes between Juliette and me, our commitment to our daughters never wavered. The challenges we faced with our oldest daughter shaped the way we viewed our lives moving forward. We knew sacrifices would need to be made, not just for her health, but for her future as well. We had no guarantees about how she would develop—how she would grow and change, whether she would ever be able to live independently, or whether she would always need our help. The uncertainty hung over us, a constant weight we had to carry, and even now, it hasn't gone away.

We started planning our lives around her needs. Everything became about ensuring she had the best possible chance at a full life, even though we didn't know what that would look like. We talked endlessly about what the future might hold, wondering how much help we'd need, and whether we'd get it. It was exhausting, not knowing, always waiting for the next obstacle to present itself. And yet, through it all,

Juliette and I stayed committed to the path we were on, even if our bond had shifted.

For a while, it felt like our love for each other had grown stronger because of the challenges we faced. Those early days, especially through the first pregnancy and up until a year after the second, were some of the closest moments we had as a couple. We were in it together, side by side, weathering the storm. But after that, things began to decline. Slowly, yes, but steadily. It's hard to admit that, but it's the truth. We didn't fall apart, not completely, but the connection that once felt unbreakable became strained under the weight of everything.

Even so, our love for our children kept us moving forward. Our younger daughter, especially, was a constant source of hope. Watching her grow, seeing her natural curiosity and strength, helped us stay grounded. And while our older daughter's challenges continued to shape our lives, it was those moments of joy with our youngest that reminded us of the good, the simple pleasures that kept us going.

I'm not sure what the future holds for us, but I do know that, no matter what, our family will always be the most important thing. And while Juliette and I may not be as close as we once were, we're still in this together—for our girls, for the life we've built, and for the love that, despite everything, still ties us all together.

Chapter 9:
Home, Work, and Life

It's funny how life takes you down paths you never quite expect. When Juliette and I first moved into her mother's home, we didn't plan on staying as long as we did. It was a temporary arrangement, something to help everyone get back on their feet after her mother's separation from her stepfather. We were a young couple, trying to figure out what came next for us, and living with her mom seemed like the best solution at the time.

In a way, it brought us closer, not just to her mom but to each other. We found ourselves relying on her in ways we hadn't anticipated.

Juliette's mom became an integral part of our lives, especially after the kids came along. She helped us through everything—caring for the children, helping with household chores, even emotional support during some of the more difficult times. There's no doubt in my mind that things would have been so much harder without her around.

As much as the idea of living with a parent felt strange to me initially, it became clear that we needed her as much as she needed us. She was going through her own struggles with the separation, and in some ways, our presence gave her a sense of stability, something to focus on besides the difficulties of her own life. We bought the stepfather's share of the house not long after that, which was a huge decision for us. It was a mutual choice, but the kids were the main factor that drove us toward it.

Looking back now, I can see that this decision—buying a share of the house—was rooted in a desire for permanence, something solid we could hold onto in a world that felt ever-shifting. The house itself had a lot of meaning for Juliette and her mom. They had shared many years there before the separation, and even though the circumstances had changed, there was a feeling of home attached to it that they weren't ready to let go of.

So, when the opportunity arose to buy the share from her stepfather, it felt like the right move, even if it was a bit uncomfortable for me at first.

At the time, we were living in the bachelor suite—a small, separate part of the house that felt a little like its own world. It wasn't ideal, and I remember feeling uneasy for the first few months. I knew Juliette's mom meant well by offering the switch and letting us take over the larger portion of the house, but it was still her home in many ways. I wasn't used to that dynamic, living in someone else's space.

Still, I understood the reasoning behind it. The decision wasn't just for us—it was for the kids, for their future, and for the sense of family we were trying to build.

Despite the difficulties, staying in that house wasn't all bad. In fact, in many ways, it became our first real home as a family. We had to make it our own, though, and that was where the real work began. The house itself was beautiful—spacious, with plenty of land surrounding it—but the inside felt a bit dated, especially the kitchen. It was rustic and charming, sure, but dark, and we both felt like it needed a bit of modernizing. So, we set to work on it, brightening things up and making it feel more like us.

The kitchen renovation was the first real project we took on together, and while it was exhausting at times, it also felt rewarding. We painted the walls, redid some of the fixtures, and tried to strike a balance between keeping its original charm while also making it feel a bit more contemporary. It wasn't just about making the space look nicer—it was about creating a place where we could see ourselves cooking meals for the kids, hosting family dinners, and making memories.

The renovations didn't stop with the kitchen. We made plenty of changes to the bachelor suite as well, which was more for Juliette's mom than for us. We wanted to make sure she had a space that felt comfortable and new after everything she had been through. We redid the floors, laid down fresh tiles, and gave the bedroom a complete makeover. It was a lot of work, but it felt like a necessary step in making the house feel right for all of us.

But the inside wasn't the only thing we worked on. We had nearly 180,000 square feet of land surrounding the house, which meant there was plenty to be done outdoors, too. One of the biggest projects was building a deck for the pool we bought. That was a project I took on with real excitement. There's something about working with your hands, creating something from the ground up, that makes you feel connected to the space in a deeper way.

We didn't stop there, either. We added a pergola, built a playground and a swing set for the kids, and even put up a big shed for extra storage. There was so much land to maintain—grass that needed constant cutting, trees to trim, and endless other little tasks that kept me busy. But in the end, it all felt worth it. The house, with all its imperfections and quirks, had become ours in every way that mattered. And while the challenges were many, the work we put into it brought a sense of satisfaction that's hard to describe.

Around that time, things were tough for me on a personal level as well. The idea of getting an apartment was out of the question. Financially, we were in no position to strike out on our own, and with a baby on the way, staying in the house made the most sense. But as anyone who's ever lived in close quarters with family knows, it wasn't always easy. At that time, I also lost my job.

There were times when it felt like we were just holding on, getting through each day one at a time. Dec. 8 was the day Juliette and I decided to separate. It was a hard decision, and while we made arrangements to stay in the house for a few more months, I finally left on April 1st. Leaving was tough. That house had become so intertwined with our family and our lives, but it was necessary.

As I think back on those times now, I realize how much that house—and the work we put into it—became a symbol of our family's resilience...

Living with Juliette's mother wasn't something I had ever imagined, and yet, when I look back now, it was one of the best decisions we could have made. At first, I had my reservations, thinking that living with a parent would make things complicated, that we'd lose our privacy or have too many conflicts over space and routines. But that wasn't the case at all. In fact, we found a balance, and it worked out better than I had ever expected.

We all had our boundaries, which was key. It wasn't like we were living on top of each other all the time. Juliette's mother had her part of the house, and we had ours. There was a certain respect for each other's space that made everything run smoothly. We'd have dinner together sometimes, especially on weekends, and those moments were always filled with laughter and good conversation. I think those late-night talks, the ones that stretched long into the evening, were some of the most comforting moments we had during that time. It was during those chats that we really got to know each other, sharing stories, worries, and hopes for the future.

There were times when I thought it might be tough, maybe even a bit awkward, to live with a parent again, but surprisingly, it didn't feel like that at all. There was no drama, no stepping on each other's toes, just a quiet understanding of what each of us needed. Having her there brought a sense of stability to our lives. We were going through a lot—having a baby on the way, managing finances, and navigating the future—and having her constant support made everything feel a little less overwhelming. She was always there, whether it was helping with the kids or offering advice, and I can't imagine how much harder it would have been without her.

Of course, buying a share of the house did add a new layer of responsibility. Financially, we had to be more careful. There was no room for frivolous spending, and Juliette was constantly searching for deals or specials online. We had to watch every penny, which, honestly, was something we were prepared for. We knew that taking on a larger portion of the house meant sacrifices in other areas, but it was worth it. This was a long-term decision for our family, something that would give us a home, not just for the short term, but for years to come.

And then there was the birth of our daughter. It was supposed to be a joyous occasion, and in many ways, it was, but it was also overshadowed by the chaos of the pandemic. The timing couldn't have been worse. The world was shutting down, and when we arrived at the hospital, everything was different from what we had expected. I wasn't even allowed inside while Juliette was in labor. I had to wait outside, pacing around, waiting for that phone call that would finally let me in. It was agonizing. Then, once I was inside, we were stuck in the room for the entire duration of the procedure and afterward. It felt surreal, being in the middle of one of the most significant moments of our lives while the world outside seemed to be falling apart. But in the end, all that mattered was that our daughter was healthy, and we were together as a family.

Living with Juliette's mother during that time made us reconsider a lot of our plans. Initially, when we moved into the bachelor suite, it was supposed to be temporary. The goal was to save enough money to buy our own house, something that was ours from the ground up. But when her parents separated, everything shifted. Suddenly, the idea of staying and making this place our own seemed more appealing. We had already invested so much into the house—emotionally and financially—that leaving didn't feel right anymore.

This experience, living with her mother, renovating the house, welcoming our daughter into the world—all of it changed me. Before all this, I had been alone for years, comfortable with the idea that I might never have a family of my own. I had reached a point where I wasn't expecting to meet someone, to fall in love, or to build this kind of life. But then everything changed. I learned what it meant to be part of a family, what it took to make a relationship work. I learned about compromise, commitment, and sacrifice, things that I hadn't really considered before.

This was a different kind of life than the one I had imagined for myself years ago, but it was one that I had come to embrace. Being a partner, a father, and a part of this family—it taught me so much about myself. It wasn't always easy, and there were moments when I wasn't sure if we were doing the right thing, but at the end of the day, it felt right. This house, this life we were building, it was ours. And as much as I had grown to love it, I knew that life had a way of surprising you when you least expected it.

There was a bittersweetness to it all, though, because as much as I had grown, I also knew that things were changing. Our relationship, the one Juliette and I had built, wasn't what it once was. Slowly, almost imperceptibly at first, things started to shift. We weren't as close as we had been in the beginning. There were cracks, little ones, but they were there, and over time, they became harder to ignore.

But that's a story for later. For now, what mattered was that we had built something together. We had created a home, raised a family, and navigated through some of the hardest challenges life could throw at us. And while I didn't know what the future would hold, I knew that this experience—living in that house, with Juliette's mother, raising our children—had changed me in ways I couldn't have anticipated.

Chapter 10:
The Strains of Change

It started as an opportunity, one that seemed too good to pass up. The chance to move up in my career, to secure a better salary, and to create a stable future for my family. It wasn't just for me; I thought I was helping her, Juliette, too. I convinced my boss at the time that she could take over my position—that she had the skills, the knowledge, the drive. They gave her a shot. And for a while, I believed everything would be fine. We had always worked well together. Our partnership felt unshakable, both in work and in life.

But life has a way of changing its course in ways you can't predict, and that's exactly what happened to us.

At first, the changes seemed small. My new job meant longer hours, coming home a bit later. Juliette, now managing her own role, had to pick up the kids more often. We still spent time together, but there was a shift. It was subtle, barely noticeable, like the slow stretching of a thread that holds two people together. And yet, it was there. I didn't realize it back then, but we were beginning to drift apart, not because we stopped caring, but because life was pulling us in different directions.

We had always communicated well at work. There was something seamless about the way we collaborated. But at home, that harmony seemed to fade. Our conversations grew fewer, more surface-level. I didn't understand why. It felt strange—how could we talk so effortlessly when working, but stumble when it came to the matters that truly mattered?

Looking back, I see now that stress was silently building. It was her first management position, and I could sense the pressure weighing on her. I tried to support her, to tell her I was there. I offered to coach her, to be her safety net, but I didn't realize that maybe that's not what she needed. Maybe she needed me to listen more, to be present in ways that I wasn't.

Then came the night that changed everything. She had been distant for some time, but I chalked it up to the new responsibilities, to work stress. I tried to ignore the sinking feeling in my gut. But that night, when I asked her if something was wrong, I saw it in her eyes—sadness mixed with anger, frustration. And then the words came out, the ones I had been dreading: "I don't think I love you anymore."

I was crushed, shattered. My world broke in an instant. The anger, the sadness, the confusion—it all hit me at once. I had no idea it had come to this. I felt blindsided, like I had been living in a world where I thought we were okay, only to find out that she had been miles ahead in making the decision to leave.

I remember trying to fix things, scrambling to hold on. I did everything I could think of—helping more around the house, trying to be more present—but nothing worked. It was as if the door had already closed, and I was standing outside, pleading to be let back in. She told me I'd have to do a lot to change her mind, but I didn't even know what I needed to change. I felt lost.

The decision to separate wasn't mutual—it was hers. I wanted to fight for us, for the life we had built, but she had already moved on, emotionally if not physically. I was left trying to understand how it all unraveled, how we went from being a team to being strangers.

The days that followed were the hardest of my life. I was broken, my heart torn apart by the weight of her words. I thought I would spend my life with her, that we were solid, unshakable. I couldn't comprehend how we had reached this point. And yet, there I was, left to pick up the pieces of a life that no longer felt whole.

As time went on, I began to see my own faults. I was physically there, yes, but emotionally? I was absent. I had been so caught up in work, in providing, that I hadn't realized I was neglecting the most important thing—our connection. I wish I had seen it sooner. Maybe then things would have been different.

I learned something through this heartbreak: just because you think everything is fine, doesn't mean the other person feels the same. Relationships require attention, effort, and most of all, presence. I regret being "absent in my presence," and I'll never make that mistake again. I thought we were invincible, that nothing could tear us apart, but I was wrong.

This experience changed me. It changed my outlook on relationships, on love, on life. It made me more aware, more attentive to the people I care about. I'm still healing—almost a year has passed, and I haven't met anyone new. But I've found strength in myself, in rebuilding my life. I bought a new house, started new job challenges, and most importantly, I focused on being there for my girls.

The separation was devastating, but it didn't break me. I stayed positive, telling myself that I could get through it, that I would find happiness again. And slowly, I did. The pain is still there, lingering in the background, but I've learned to push through it. To keep going, for myself and for my daughters.

I am writing this book not just to find answers, but to heal. And in a way, it has helped. Juliette and I communicate better now. As she told me just a few days ago, "If we couldn't make our relationship work, we have to be the best parents for our children." That's our new focus—our kids, and giving them the best life we can, even if we aren't together anymore.

To anyone going through something similar, my words to you are simple: keep your head up. Amazing things can happen, even after the darkest moments. You just have to keep pushing forward, to find strength in the little moments, and to never lose hope.

Epilogue

I remember the day Juliette and I separated like it was yesterday, even though it came in the most understated way, with no explosive arguments or final showdown. It was quiet—too quiet. The signs had been there, subtle but growing louder in hindsight. I felt choked with sadness, anger, and confusion, like waves crashing into each other inside me, leaving me drowning. It was like reaching for something just as it slips through your fingers—grasping only emptiness where there was once warmth.

For months after she left, I couldn't shake the feeling that maybe it was just a phase, that we would find our way back to each other. But that Mother's Day, when I sent her flowers, and she told me so definitively, "It's over. No turning back," it finally shattered any hope I'd held onto. Her words were like a door slamming shut, echoing in my mind. I knew I had to stop hoping, to let go for my own sake, and for the kids. Still, even today, I can't say that the love just vanished. She was the love of my life—or at least, I thought so—and those feelings don't disappear just because you tell them to.

There was one time when I thought maybe we could talk things out, so I wrote her a letter. It wasn't anything fancy—just a reply to the list she'd given me, of all the things she needed from me, all the ways I'd fallen short. Looking back, there were things on that list that I could have changed, things I would have been willing to change. But it was already too late. She had made up her mind. I found out later that she had been thinking about leaving for over a year but hadn't felt confident enough to make the leap until she secured that big job with a decent salary. It was as if she was waiting for the right moment to be self-sufficient, and once she had it, she walked away.

That letter didn't bring closure. If anything, it deepened the hurt, making me feel like I hadn't been enough. That's a hard thing to come to terms with—the idea that despite everything, you weren't what someone else needed. It felt like I was watching a part of myself die, and it took a long time to put that part to rest.

These days, I live alone in a little house about 45 minutes away. It's nothing special, but I'm slowly fixing it up, piece by piece, giving it some life. I didn't jump into another relationship because, honestly, I wasn't ready. The house, the kids, and my work kept me busy, filling the empty hours and numbing the pain just a little. I poured myself into renovating each room, as if, by rebuilding my surroundings, I could rebuild myself. It's been nearly a year now, and maybe, just maybe, I'm ready to meet someone new. I feel like I could let someone in, but this time, I know I need to be more present—not just physically but emotionally. It's a tough thing to figure out.

My kids...not seeing them every day—that's been the hardest part. There's a quiet ache when I wake up, and they're not there, just silence where their laughter used to be. At first, it felt unbearable, a hollow pain I couldn't escape. But over time, I've found a way to cope. I see them as often as I can, and my plan has always been to renovate and sell this house, so I can eventually buy a place closer to them. It's the driving force behind every nail I hammer, every wall I paint. I want to be closer, to make the distance just a little smaller.

This experience has changed me in ways I never imagined. I thought I was strong before, but this broke me in ways I didn't see coming. Yet, somehow, in that brokenness, I found a new strength. I learned that when you set your mind to something, when you have no choice but to survive, you can dig up a resilience you didn't know existed. I feel stronger now, not invincible, but solid, grounded. If I could survive this, I can survive anything.

As for love, I haven't given up on it. I've realized that love needs care and attention, like a flower. If you water it, tend to it, nurture it, it can last. But ignore it, and it withers before you even notice. I wasn't always there when Juliette needed me; I see that now, and I'm learning from it.

Juliette left a permanent mark on my life. Before her, I never thought about having kids; they just weren't in the picture. But with her, that changed. We faced some of the scariest moments together, especially during the first pregnancy. It bonded us in a way I thought could never be undone. Even though things ended badly, I'll always care about her because she gave me something priceless—our children.

For anyone else walking this path of love, loss, and trying to find solid ground again, I would say this: if there's something worth fighting for, fight as hard as you can. But if it's clear that nothing more can be done, try to let go, no matter how much it hurts. Acceptance doesn't mean the pain disappears, but it does mean that, eventually, you'll find the strength to move forward. And when you do, you'll realize that the path is wide open again, ready for whatever comes next.

www.ingramcontent.com/pod-product-compliance
Lightning Source LLC
Chambersburg PA
CBHW051234120626
46547CB00013B/1641